I0408385

Calisthenics for Beginners:
10 Steps to Build Your Own Bodyweight Training Program

Combine the Best Bodyweight Exercises in Ways that Allow You to get an Incredibly Effective Street Workout

Timothy Morrison

Table of Contents

Introduction

The word calisthenics comes from the ancient Greek words kalos (κάλλος),
which means "beauty", and sthenos (σθένος), meaning "strength".
It is the art of using one's body weight and qualities of inertia
as a means to develop one's physique.

Wikipedia

Calisthenics has its origin in ancient times. Obviously, it was a sufficient component of warrior's and athlete's training since those old times. All basic bodyweight exercises like push-ups, squats, and pull-ups are as aged as man's first try at becoming stronger by virtue of physical training.

And ironically, Calisthenics also is one of the **newest** trends in the fitness world. Term 'Calisthenics' is closely connected with 'street workout.' There are few worldwide sports organizations like the World Street Workout & Calisthenics Federation (WSWCF) and World Calisthenics Organization (WCO). Rules for competitions with judging criteria and weight categories are created too.

As we see generally, Calisthenics is associated with bodyweight strength training and gymnastic tricks on an overhand bar and parallel bars.

However, I believe that Calisthenics is something much wider than that. It is closer to the physical development term. Besides the strength, you should develop your endurance, your coordination, your dexterity, your balance.

Also, bodyweight exercise is an umbrella term for some disciplines that use gravity and inertia of body as a primary form of resistance. For instance, yoga and gymnastics are well known and very popular disciplines. Parkour is another example that has increased in popularity of late. Some experts consider cardiovascular exercise like running to be forms of bodyweight exercise too.

You are the person who defines the goals and builds your own system of training. Changing with time your aims and priorities is a quite natural way of your physical development. You also could choose a set of skills which is a key factor in your favorite sport and work on it.

Don't afraid to try something new and define what works for you. The dogmatic approach doesn't work well in long term perspective. The best training plan is the one you are going to follow up.

The more you train in new ways and angles, the easier it becomes to gain new skills. On the other hand, you need some time and efforts to progress in one particular direction. The balance between your goals and your time plus efforts is a key factor here. You should remember that.

Step 1: Choose the Right Strength Training Exercises According to Your Fitness Level.

As we admitted previously, bodyweight exercises are known for centuries if not longer. However, the ways these exercises are performed are also developing rapidly. Training schemes, principles, and programs now draw heavily from weightlifting bodybuilding which is a mainstream way to add strength and gain muscle. The great thing about weight lifting and bodyweight training is that you don't have to pick one or the other. Mix up the type of stimulation. It's a good way to shock your muscles into new growth incessantly.

Bodyweight exercises imitate real life moves. You probably have heard a "functional training" term. So you learn to be strong and to perform in ways you will need to in real life. That's why Calisthenics is good for conditioning for sports such as boxing or martial arts.

Basic exercises in Calisthenics are compound movements. It is convenient to divide all muscle groups to upper body muscles and lower body muscles. Upper body muscles in their turn could be split into two another groups: push and pull.

Push muscles primarily include chest, shoulders, and triceps. It is logical that main movements here are push-ups and dips. Actually, they are two variants of one movement.

Regular **push-ups** are simple and handy exercises, require nothing more than the floor beneath your feet. If you don't have access to weight-training equipment, you still can perform push-ups. The proper form of push-ups provides the load for your entire core, not just your upper body.

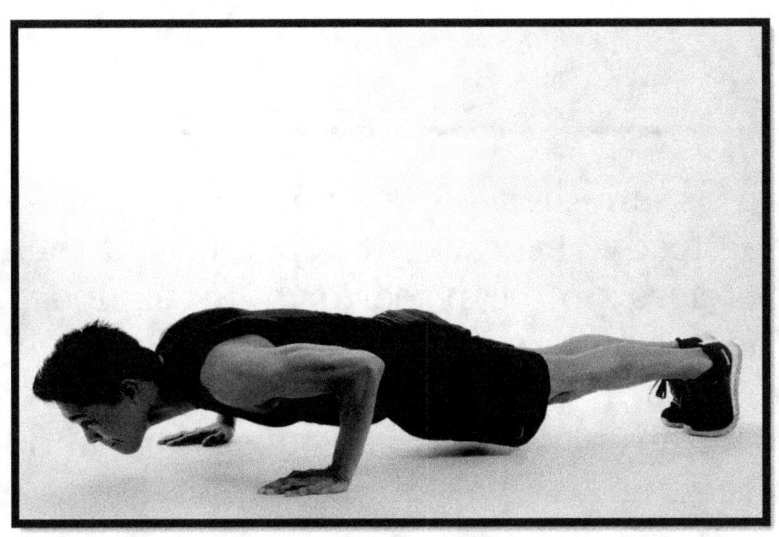

There is a huge number of push-ups variants with different levels of difficulty. Most challenging are one hand push-ups and headstand push-ups. You'll need not only a sufficient level of strength but also a significant amount of stability for performing headstand push-ups. One hand push-ups force you to engage your lats, opposite-side leg, lower back, and glutes.

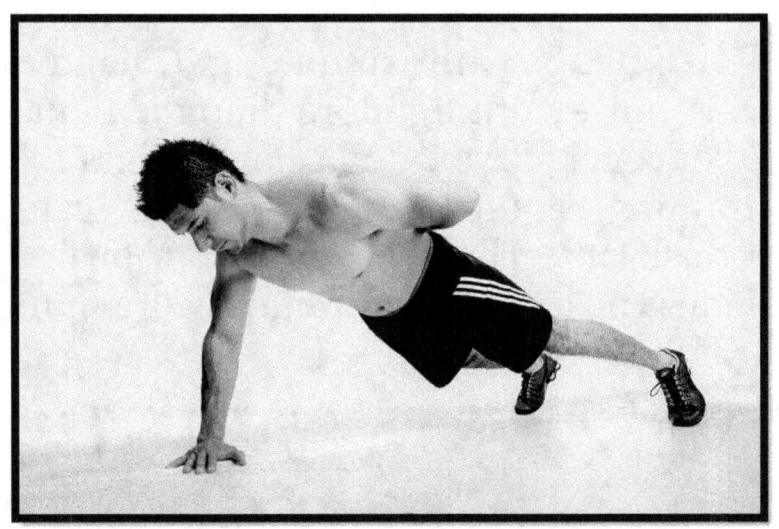

The **dip** is another old-school, simple-yet-brutally-effective exercise. It is just one of the best exercises you can perform to explode your chest, shoulders, and triceps. Parallel bar dips train your push muscles in an entirely different angle than push-ups and bench pressing.

You also could try ring dips. Such form requires much more stability to perform. It's one of the harder variations you can do.

We are not focused on details of exercise's technique in this book. Training videos work perfectly, so I have added some links to YouTube playlists.

Push muscles exercises on YouTube:
https://goo.gl/TRisUP

Pull muscles primarily include back and biceps. Apparently, this body part is trained by **pull-ups**. Pull-up is a gold standard exercise for back training. No exercise can equal pull-ups for effectiveness in building strength and growth of your back. It is the fact that in gyms many people prefer to use pull-down machines than pull-ups. Not surprisingly, many gym-goers are unable of doing even one clean pull-up. Invest your time and efforts to be strong at pull-ups. It will develop real strength, muscle mass, and explosiveness.

There is also a wide variety of different ways to execute pull-ups. For example, you can use wide or close grip. Underhand grip is another option here.

A true one-arm pull-up is also possible. It is tough, much harder than mentioned above one hand push-ups.

Pull muscles exercises on YouTube:
https://goo.gl/XMMEEY

Lower body primarily includes quadriceps, glutes, and calves. Some of these muscles are the biggest and most powerful in your body. So, it could be difficult to build tremendous strength in your lower body without weights. However, if extremely developed leg muscles are not paramount to you, then do not worry about it. Bodyweight squats, lunges and different kinds of jumps work well here.

And, of course, one leg **pistol squats** come to mind as a most challenging variant. As some others Calisthenics exercise pistol develops the perfect combination of power, balance, coordination, and flexibility.

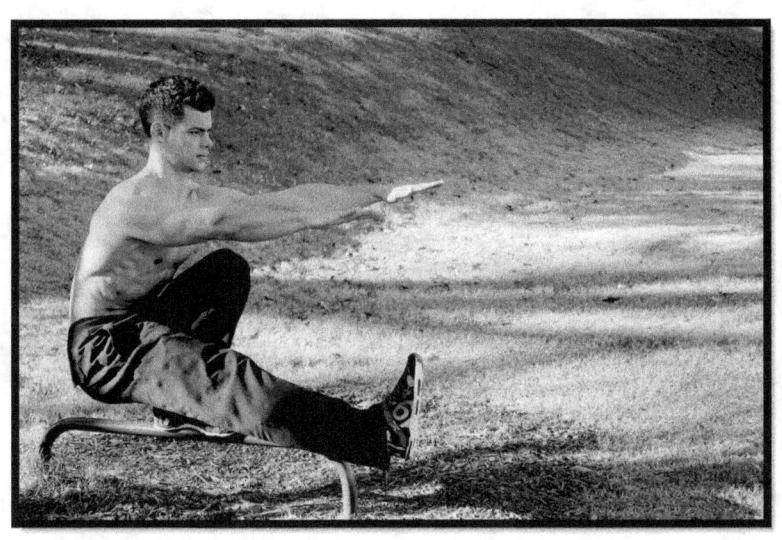

Leg exercises on YouTube:
https://goo.gl/R2Tnu0

Beyond that, abs are trained by leg raising, sit-ups, crunches.

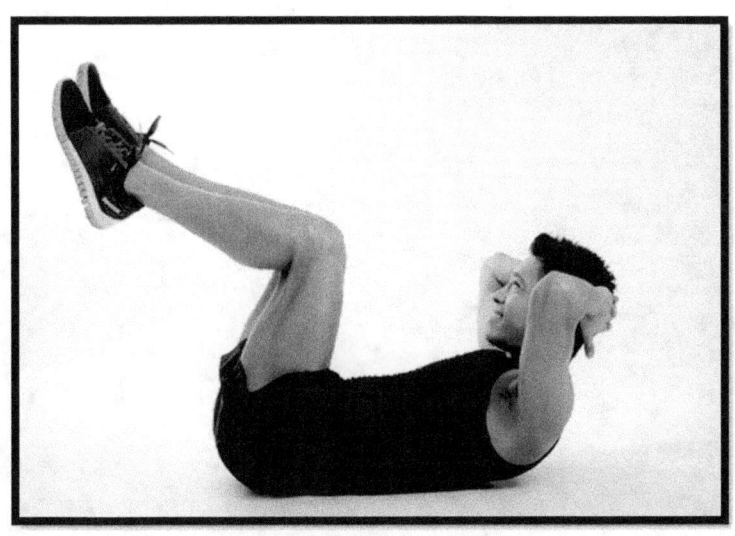

Plank works excellent for the whole core. A well-developed core shows both power and health. The hyperextension on the ground keeps in tone your low back.

Core exercises on YouTube: https://goo.gl/k5dba2

You Can't Do Pull-ups? Then This Chapter is for You!

So, pull-ups are hard. Surely, you might be not very good at them, especially, if you're just started. Then it is reasonable to consider making your back exercises a priority number 1 in your training plan. There are few exercises which are perfect precursors to regular pull ups. It's also a good cause to learn some of the hypertrophy training principles.

1.   Horizontal pull-ups are also known under name 'reverse push-ups.' This variation is a lot easier since your weight is on the floor mostly. Still, it's a good first step to the vertical, usual pull-up.

An isometric exercise is a form of exercise involving the static contraction of a muscle without any visible movement in the angle of the joint. The term "isometric" combines the Greek words "Isos" (equal) and "metria" (measuring), meaning that in these exercises the length of the muscle and the angle of the joint do not change, though contraction strength may be varied.

2.   Timed hang or 'dead hang' is an isometric exercise. Hang with straight arms and feet of the ground for 10-30 seconds or as long as you can. Focus on keeping your shoulders in the packed position. Don't let them up around your neck. You can use different grip variations in following sets.

3.   The static hold is also hanging on the bar but this time on the top movement of the pull-up. You hold that flexed position for 10-30 seconds or as long as you can.

A negative repetition (negative rep) is the repetition of a technique in weightlifting in which the lifter performs the eccentric phase of a lift. Instead of pressing the weight up slowly, in proper form, a spotter generally aids in the concentric, or lifting, portion of the repetition while the lifter slowly performs the eccentric phase for 3–6 seconds. Negative reps are used to improve both muscular strength and power.

4.   Negative pull-ups are half pull-ups. From the top position, you lower yourself down slowly, in-control. How to set up that top position? There are a set of options. You can use a bench, or a box, or a chair. You can

jump above the pull bar or use a help of your training partner.

Partial reps, as the name implies, involves movement through only part of the normal path of an exercise. Partial reps can be performed with heavier weights. Usually, only the easiest part of the repetition is attempted.

5.   Partial pull-ups involve only partial amplitude – at the top or the bottom of a movement. Top-partial pull-ups are my favorite, but you should try both variants. You also can do partial reps after complete pull-ups, when you can't do any more full reps.

As you can see, pull-ups mastering is all about progressions. I mean a chain of exercises that get progressively more difficult until you rich your goal. And off cause you can't do pull-ups if you don't practice pull-ups. So, it's up to you.

Pull-up tips for beginners on YouTube: https://goo.gl/VpXGlp

Step 2: Apply Bodybuilding Training Principles to Your Workout.

In the previous chapter we have considered such training principles as negatives, partial reps, and isometric tension. There are many other advanced techniques. Most of them were gathered and honed by Joe Weider, the father of modern bodybuilding.

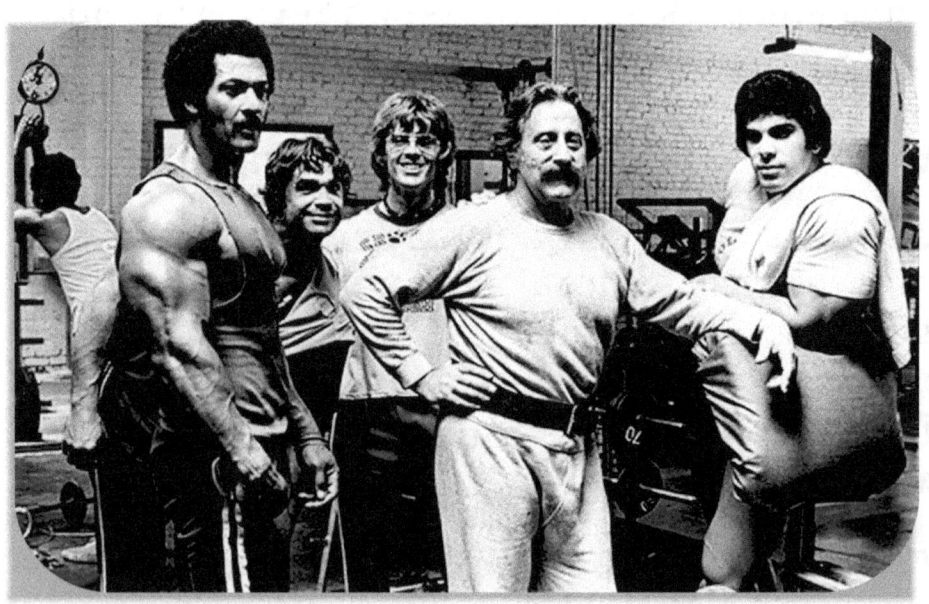

Some of that principles work to bodyweight training perfectly.

Push-pull supersets pair exercises for opposing body parts in sequence without rest.

In bodybuilding gyms, this method is especially popular when applied to arm training. Arnold used supersets to his chest-back workout mostly. You can do both by combination pull-ups and dips. You allow your chest and triceps to rehab while your back and biceps are working, and vice versa. So, you can do more repetition in each set. As a result, you'll get a sizable pumping, and that visual benefit is superb motivation. You also can do a lot of work in short time. On the hormonal level, push-pull superset leads to a spike of HGH, which is responsible for muscle growth and fat loss.

Supersets of exercises for the same body part are much more exhausting. For example, you can combine dips with push-ups. Another variant is pull-ups with 'reverse push-ups.' Regular squats after pistol squats are also good for your legs.

Forced reps are repetition after your muscular failure. You will need a training partner who provides enough help to complete the set. It's a classic thing with pull-ups. It is also applicable with dips.

The **rest-pause** method could be implemented in two options.

1.   You take your set to failure, then rest for 10-20 seconds, and continue to do reps till you reach failure once more. Repeat this trick 2-3 times per set and you will get more reps in a given exercise.

2.   You choose an exercise that only allows you to get 3-5 repetitions. You do one rep, rest 15 seconds, and perform another rep. Your goal is 4-6 repetitions, which form one rest-pause set. This variant is effective at increasing muscle strength.

Step 3: Learn About Full-body Workout and Split Training Routine.

How often should you do your strength training? Well, the answer depends on too many factors. I like to train each muscle group twice a week. One of the workouts is hard, and another is light.

On the hard training, I try to push my limits by increasing number of reps or/and sets. Using some of the principles described in the previous chapter is possible too.

The light training is just refreshing for muscles, and you don't need many sets and reps. You should focus on proper technique instead. You can also try some new exercise or method during your light training.

For example, my previous hard and light training plans for pull muscles look like:

Monday, hard training.

1.   Wide-grip pull-ups, 5 sets of 10 reps.

Usually, the last set is challenging one. I can do 7 to 8 repetitions before reaching failure. Then I do from 1 to 3 forced reps. Use the box to help yourself to bring your chin over the bar.

2. Wide-grip reverse push-ups on the low horizontal bar, 2 sets of 20 reps.

Keep the negative phase of movement lasted twice as the positive one.

3. Dead hang, one set for as long as possible.

I've found that my grip is the weak link in the chain of pull muscles. Train your forearms to progress faster in pull-ups.

Thursday, light training.

1. Middle-grip pull-ups, 3 sets of 5 reps.

Focus on the strict technique of your movements. Besides, my back and biceps are still in pain after the hard training on Monday.

2. Close-grip chin-ups, 3 sets of 5 reps.

I like this form with the accent on my biceps. Probably, I'll include chin-ups in my hard training later.

Full body workout combines exercises like push-ups, pull-ups, basic core work, and squats. This style of training twice per week can build strength without sacrificing hours to the gym. Full body is one of the oldest and well-known training plans.

	Monday (Tuesday)	Thursday (Friday)
Push muscles	HARD	LIGHT
Pull muscles	LIGHT	HARD
Legs	HARD	LIGHT
Core	LIGHT	HARD

You train all your muscles per workout; you have enough time for recovery. Full body scheme works quite well any goal like increasing strength, building muscle, losing fat.

Upper-lower body training split is the next level. You are training four times per week now: two upper body workouts and two lower body workouts. You do all chosen kinds of pull-ups, dips, and push-ups on your upper body workout. Lower body workout includes squats, jumps, exercises for your core and lower back. Upper-lower body split allows you to spend more time and efforts on every muscle group. Mentioned above push-pull supersets fit perfectly. You still train each muscle group twice a week. And you still mix hard and light training days.

	Push muscles	Pull muscles	Legs	Core
Sunday				
Monday	LIGHT	HARD		
Tuesday			HARD	LIGHT
Wednesday				
Thursday	HARD	LIGHT		
Friday			LIGHT	HARD
Saturday				

Here is an example of an upper-lower body split training plan. To perform a superset, execute exercises with the same digit but different letter designation back to back, without rest between them. Rest interval between supersets is 60 seconds.

Monday: pull hard, push light.

1A. Wide-grip pull-ups, 5 sets of 12 reps.

1B. Pike push-ups, 5 sets of 10 reps.

2A. Close-grip, chin-ups, 3 sets of 8 reps.

2B. Dips on bench, 3 sets of 8 reps.

Tuesday: legs hard, core light.

1.   Pistol squats, 5 sets of 12 reps.

2.   Jump squats, 4 sets of 20 reps

3A. Crunches, 3 sets of 25 reps

3B. Reverse crunches, 3 sets of 25 reps.

Thursday: push hard, pull light

1A. Dips on parallel bars, 5 sets of 15 reps

1B. Horizontal pull-ups, 5 sets of 15 reps.

2A. Knuckle push-ups, 3 sets of 20 reps.

2B. Dead hang, 3 sets. Try last for 60 seconds each set.

Friday: core hard, legs light.

1.   Legs raises on pull-up bar, 5sets of 15 reps.

2A. High crunches, 3 sets of 20 reps.

2B. Floor hyperextensions, 3 sets of 20 reps.

3.   Plank, for 60 seconds.

4A. Lunges, 5 sets of 15 reps.

4B. Squats, 5 sets of 20 reps.

Don't forget to change exercise with time. Try new variants on your light days. Then implement them in your hard training.

Pull-push-legs split provides even more focus for every muscle group of yours. Pulling muscles, pushing muscles, and legs are trained separately on their own workout day. There are six workouts in a week. And still, every muscle group is worked roughly twice per week and allowed roughly 72 hours to rehab.

Step 4: Improve Your Cardiovascular Fitness.

Cardio also is known as aerobic exercise is a physical activity that is long, repetitive, and depends mostly on the aerobic metabolism. Cardio in some way is opposite to anaerobic (strength) training. The difference is in duration and intensity of work. For instance, jogging is a cardio drill, though sprinting is an anaerobic exercise.

Several studies show us that cardio training can elevate results of strength training. With cardiovascular exercises, you will get greater gains! For instance, cardio can boost your work capacity during bodyweight strength workout; enhance your recovery between sessions, and improve your muscular physique. As we know, in order to burn fat and slim down, some amount of cardio training will need to be done.

Systematic prolonged training stimulates the growth of new blood vessels in your muscles. As a result, your muscle tissue gets more oxygen, macro- and micronutrients, vitamins, and therefore repairs faster.

It is also possible to strengthen your heart with regular cardio exercise. Indeed, doing aerobic exercises over the years, you can develop your heart in volume. And heart's work becomes more efficient in this case.

Good aerobic workout makes you feel like a totally new person. You know that feeling of lightness and freedom, and your mind becomes clear. After forty minutes of intense cardio training, your body starts to regenerate your nerve cells. New neurons begin to appear too. Surprisingly, the old and well-known expression 'nerve cells do not regenerate' doesn't work for you anymore.

In order to achieve the best possible result of training, you need to pick an exercise that fit your purpose. And again the best choice is the one you are going to stick with. Surely, you can change your exercises depending on the target and mood. The basic rule here is 'don't give up training.' If you want to have a stable and long-term effect, you must regularly train throughout the life. Without training sessions, all health benefits will disappear in a few weeks.

Cardio training is not just about running and rope skipping; the same old cardio gets boring very quickly. Cardio training includes numerous different exercises. The biggest part of them is performed chiefly by the leg muscles. However, there are some exceptions. What is your favorite sport to watch? Which is your favorite sport to play? The more you train your muscles and brain in new and foreign ways, the easier it becomes to master new skills. Basketball, tennis, baseball, and football places far greater demands on coordination, balance, and flexibility than strength training alone does.

If you like boxing and other martial arts you should take a look at Tae Bo. This fitness system was invented and developed by Billy Blanks. Tae Bo combines aerobic exercises, kicks, and punches. Actually, the name 'Tae Bo' goes from taekwondo and boxing.

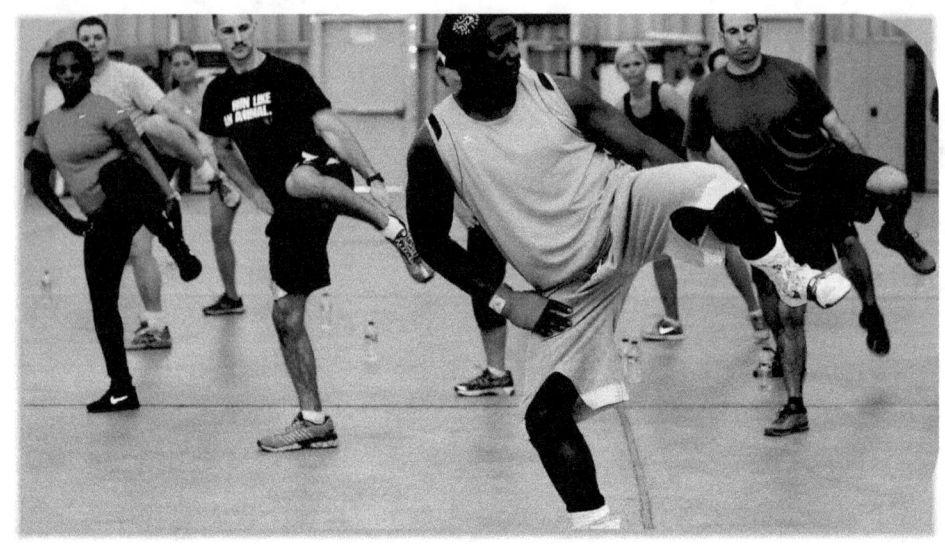

Though Tae Bo is not intended for combat or self-defense, your fight part of 'fight-or-flight' instinct could be encouraged sufficiently. Finding such a 'deep reason' creates a strong motivation for your training. The best training plan is the one you are going stick to, remember? If you enjoy what you are doing, you will progress very fast.

Personally, I've found that shadowboxing fits me just perfectly. Shadow-boxing is the practice of performing repetitive fighting movements to muscle memory. Clearly, it works well for striking techniques, not for grappling. Shadowboxing is one of the most important drills to improve technique, speed, endurance, rhythm, footwork, defense and offense, and overall fighting abilities. The primary goal here is to get used to fighting movements. This exercise is pure calisthenics as soon as you don't need any equipment. Shadowboxing is also completely harmless as there is no opponent trying to hit you.

Shadowbox according to rounds. You should plan each round before you start shadowbox. Trying to work on every aspect at once is the worst thing you can do for your progress. So, you need a goal.

If your goal is **warming-up** use shadowboxing to get warm and break a sweat. Use footwork actively, don't forget about head-movement, and throw punches. Keep your body in motion. Move designedly in, out, and around.

Shadowboxing is the best of acquiring proper **technique**. This exercise should be used to habituate each new move like a punch, defensive tech, or footwork. Repetitions are necessary but only after you know that you are doing right. I mean, you need feedback. This is where having someone more experienced in boxing helps. Also, it is a good idea to practice in front of a full-length mirror so that the movements can be watched for correct form.

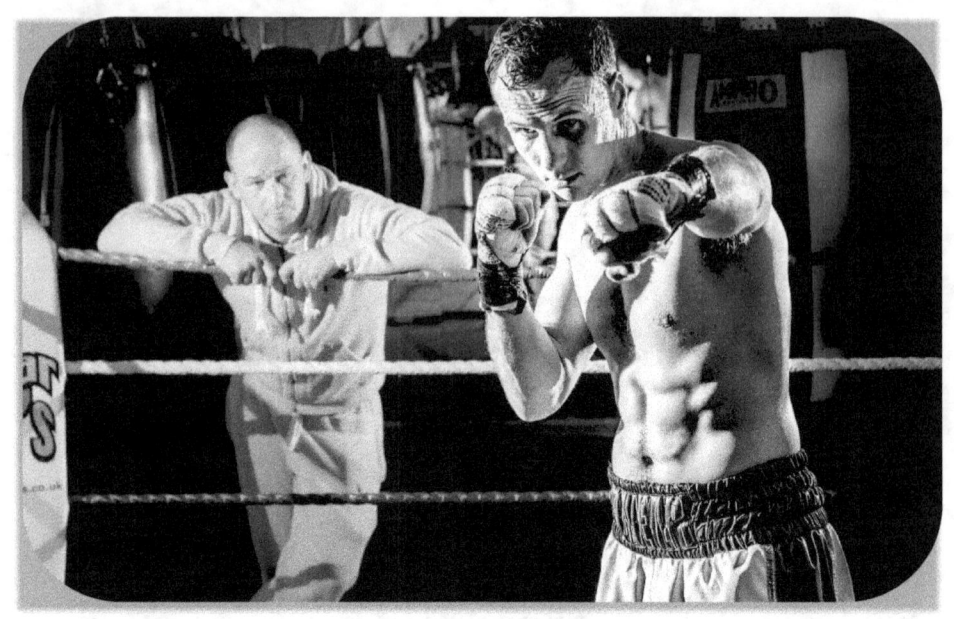

One more reason to shadowbox is developing your **coordination** and **balance**. Every time you are training you work on developing new mind-muscle connections. Eventually, during a real fight or intense sparring, this is what you will rely on. Your rival always tries to make you miss, and in every miss you get off-balanced. Shadowboxing is the perfect method to train the supporting muscles to counteract the momentum generated in every your attack. After all, with well developed stabilizing muscles and coordination, you can throw nice combos of powerful shots while maintaining balanced.

Simulating actual actions used in a fight will **condition** your hand and leg endurance. You also can work on your **rhythm** while shadowboxing by making many punches, defenses, and footwork. Throwing punches with full extension and power all the time is not a very good idea for your joint health. So sometimes it is ok to minimize your hand movements. Let's focus on torso rotation over arm extension, and your joints will thank you for it. Explosive footwork and head movement will provide sufficient level of intensity.

Shadowboxing is a mental exercise also. You could go into every round with focus on implementing specific **strategies**. And yes, strategies are needed even for something as primary as fighting. Shadowboxing is an excellent opportunity to work out a strategy to beat your opponent. Then you master new technical things like punch combinations to fulfill this plan. Punches are often labeled with digits to simplify training process. There are typical numbers associated with every punch in boxing:

1 – jab

2 –right straight (cross)

3 – left hook

4 – right hook (overhand)

5 – left uppercut

6 – right uppercut

Body shots are just called as 'body'. Basic punching combinations are:

1-2 with variations (1 – 2body,   1body – 2)

1 – 2 – 3   (1 – 2body – 3,   1 – 2 – 3body, 1body – 2 – 3)

1 – 1 – 2   (1 – 1 – 2body,   1 – 1body – 2, 1body – 1 – 2)

1 – 2 – 1   (1body – 2 – 1,   1 – 2body – 1)

1 – 2 – 3 – 2   (1 – 2body – 3 – 2, 1body – 2 – 3 – 2)

Master the standard punch combo. Then try advanced or/and start creating your own. Surely, with the kicks, elbows, and knees in your arsenal, you will have an even much wider diversity of your training routine. *Examples of shadowboxing routines on YouTube: https://goo.gl/TYD08q*

Shadowboxing also could be substituted in place of an aerobic or anaerobic conditioning session, with the duration and intensity reflecting a jogging for long distance or set of sprints.

Step 5: Don't Forget About Recovery.

The whole training process and its benefits are all about keeping the balance between stress and recovery. Due to strength exercise execution, you break some part of your muscle tissue down. After a workout, your muscle fibers repair themselves and come back bigger and stronger than they were before. As you can see, the scheme of the whole process is pretty simple. The tricky part is to define how much time you need to recover efficiently. Because, if you tax the same muscles every day heavily, you aren't them the time they need to rehab. As a result, you'll get overtraining. Usual signals of overtraining are decreased performance, elevated blood pressure, decreased immunity, disturbed sleep.

By performing hard-light workout scheme and training splits, you train each muscle group enough to add strength, but not so much that you need to rest for too many days between each strength workout. Plus, you have time to enjoy your cardio training on a more recreational basis. Such an active recovery will provide the blood flowing, more nutrients, and oxygen to those sore, torn muscles. Naturally, this will accelerate the process of recovery.

To determine adequate rest between workouts you should consider many different factors. Your age could be a factor and how intensely you train, how often you work out, and the duration of exercise.

So, you will listen to your body and change your schedule when you need. For example, if you feel sore for hard-day strengthen workout, perform cardio or light-day session. Yes, light training is one of the best ways to resolve muscle soreness. This phenomenon is well known as 'repeated-bout effect.'

Or, if you feel exhausted all of the time, you may need to take one more day off. Probably, you like many people tend to over-train, which can delay your progress. You should keep symptoms of overtraining at bay. It's all about maintaining balance, remember?

Step 6: Sleep Better, Rehab Faster.

The best training routine, diet and supplement plan will not compensate for poor quality sleep. Sleep just might be the most important element of your training schedule. Often the key to winning is the quality and amount of sleep you get. You need at least eight hours of quality sleep per night. Elite athletes are known to sleep ten hours a night and nap throughout the day between workouts to maintain their endurance. 'Get enough for you' is the best practical recommendation here.

Little sleep means little results because without adequate rest your body will fail to adapt. Of course, you can be sleep deprived from time to time. However, if it is a permanent situation, it will have an enormous impact on your training results. Also, getting too little sleep accumulates a so-called 'sleep debt.' We couldn't adapt to getting less sleep than we need, so your body will 'pay back,' eventually.

Sleep has a profound effect on physical well-being and every part of our life. Up to 70% of daily human growth hormone secretion is naturally released under conditions of sleep. This hormone stimulates fat burning, muscle growth, and repair. Thus the more sleep you get, the faster your body will heal and recover from exercise.

Your exercise can help your sleep; it is kind of synergy effect. However, sometimes it is hard to get a good night of sleep. The following simple rules can assist in getting that proper night rest.

Complete your training at least four hours before going to bed. Avoid caffeine and other stimulants within those four hours too. Don't eat large meals just before bedtime, small snacks are allowed.

Go to bed and wake up at the consistent times every day.

Do not watch TV in bed, instead make some sleep routine. Shut off electronics and write in a diary. Take a warm bath. Minimize light and noise, meditate.

Any other things that relax and bring down the body are acceptable.

Step 7: Stick to a Muscle-Building Diet.

Second, the most important recovery factor is food. You should focus on proper nutrition when it comes to getting the results you want. Intensive training is an incredibly demanding job. That's why what you ingest in the minutes and hours after your workout is so critical to recovery. One of the most beneficial things you can do for your calisthenics program is a post-workout nutrition strategy.

Ingesting carbohydrates within thirty minutes of the workout is crucial to initiating muscle glycogen synthesis. Experts recommend post-workout consuming 0.5g of carbs per pound of bodyweight.

Also, most experts agree that athletes will get hoped-for benefit by consuming right dose (30g) of protein within the first-hour post-workout.

Usually, we finish a training session in some fluid deficit. Drinking 150% of the estimated fluid loss will enhance rapid and complete recovery from dehydration. Sipping fluids is preferable to drinking large amounts at one time.

If you want to gain some muscle mass, you will need an excess of calories. If you are a teenage hard-gainer, you will need to consume even more calories because your metabolism is very high. When you take in more than expanded calories, and weight is being gained, fatigue reducing becomes much more efficient. You also eat much more carbs, up to 3g per pound per day for hard-training days.

During fat loss dieting you reduce consumption of carbohydrates, as well as calories intake. Keep in mind, that cutting carbs will have an adverse impact on fatigue. So, cut the minimum you can to get still the result you need. And make sure the other recovery factors like proper training management and quality sleep are in order.

As much as possible avoid junk food in favor of eating muscle building foods like white and red meat, whole eggs, and fish.

Vegetables and fruits contain not only carbohydrates but water, vitamins, minerals, antioxidants, and fiber. Some of these nutrients affect the speed at which glucose releases into the bloodstream. That's why these products are recommended for sustained energy during the day.

Step 8: Use Periodized Training Plans for Better Results.

As we said previously, it is important to focus on one particular goal for a period of time. It is also a good intention to switch it up to a different goal at the next period. You don't want always be working towards the same goal. It's too boring, and your mind needs a change of pace in order to keep you motivated enough. At the same time, your body needs time to recover from training in a given mode.

Yes, the 'goal' is a key word here. The two most common fitness goals are building muscle and fat loss. And of course, I want to get both at once. However, you will achieve better results if you include two different periods in your training plan.

In order to perform your 'leaning out' phase, you are going to add more cardio in your program. You can start with two full-body strength workouts and four half-hour cardio sessions every week. You may also wish to make some changes in your diet. Moderation your calories and especially carbohydrates intake is a good move. You need clean sources of complex carbohydrates only, so avoid simple carbs. Timing is an important thing too. Cut down on your intake later on in the evening when your body needs less energy. Focus more on eating carbs in your breakfast and around your workout as this when you need fuel most. Be sure you are having lots of water.

In order to execute your 'gaining muscle' phase, you are going to focus on your strength workouts. I suppose four upper-lower-body split workouts and two cardio sessions a week is a good plan. You need many calories, and you should focus on clean sources of protein, carbs, and healthy fats at each meal.

How long should you stick to a particular phase? Well, I would say two to three months is an optimal duration. One excellent way to set up a training program is with seasons. Do you always try to lose fat come summer, like most people do? Then you can take this concept and build your program around it.

You are right; whole this periodization-thing looks like bodybuilders program, where they cycle periods of bulking with fat loss. Well, systematic planning of training applies in nearly all sports. Martial arts, wrestling, football, basketball, baseball, and swimming are a few that fall into this category. Actually, anyone interested in a general base of fitness, skills, and strength would, as well. These athletes would also require speed, strength endurance, hypertrophy, and aerobic endurance, to varying proportions. Each of these requires a special form of training and some conflict to the others. The common goal is preparation for the most important competition of the year. There are longer cycles for the Olympian, being four and eight years. Another example is the career plan which is usually only considered for professional athletes.

Step 9: Set SMART Fitness Goals.

I couldn't stress enough the importance of having goals. Next crucial point in creating your bodyweight training program that will work best for you is figuring out what your fitness goal is. Whether you want to burn fat, increase strength or just look great naked adopting your training regimen plays a significant role.

Set goals for your nearest training cycle and apply the SMART criteria to each of your goals.

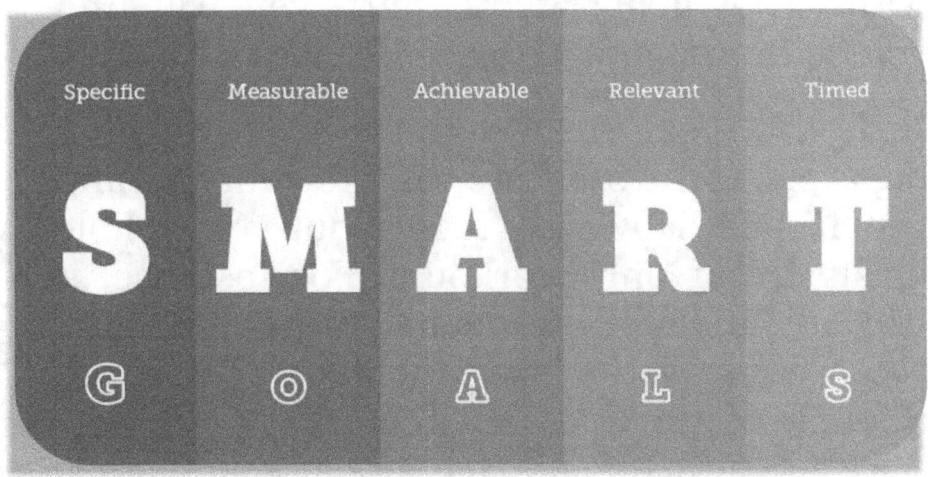

Specific aim declares exactly what you want to accomplish. For example, make a goal of 'performing ten reps of pistol squats' rather than 'increasing leg strength.'

Measurability allows you to track the progress and measure the outcome. How much muscle are you planning to gain? Put some numbers in your goal. These numbers could define exercise repetitions, fat percentage, waist to chest ratio, weight to gain, and so on.

Attainable goal is reasonable enough to be accomplished. If you have never done a single pull-up before, wanting to perform fifteen reps of regular pull-ups within a month is not an attainable goal. Obviously, you should always take into account your experience with certain exercise. Furthermore, after success with easier goals at the start, you will find yourself more motivated.

Relevant goal meets your need. If you want big arms, focus on exercises like chin-ups and bench dips. However, it is about your whole lifestyle, not only workouts. For instance, if you are unwilling to change your diet, then you can't expect to lose weight significantly in a couple of months.

Timed goal provides a time limit. It will establish a sense of urgency. Also, having a deadline will motivate you to stick to your program when you feel like slacking off.

Eventually, setting a time limit will let you know whether or not you workout routine is effective as your progress.

Setting SMART goals do not have to be difficult, so let's give it a try. The summer is coming, and off course, I want six packs. I will know that I've achieved my purpose when I see a six-pack in the mirror. In order to realize my goal, I need to reduce body fat by five percent. I will do two strengthen workouts and four cardio sessions a week for the next two months. And I will increase my result in 'leg raises on bar' exercise by ten repetitions at the end of this cycle. I will cut my daily intake by 500 calories. I will avoid all kinds of sweetness and processed food. I will eat complex carbohydrates before and after my workouts. I won't drink a beer and sweet beverages, only plain water. I will stick to this regimen for the next two months.

It looks like I get a kit of goals, isn't it? Well, it happens when you want just to get six packs.

Step 10: Track Your Progress Using a Training Diary.

A training diary is one of the best tools you can use for achieving your goals; it's an important key to success. At its most basic minimum, this is a written record of exercises and repetitions for every set you do. Also, record the quality of your repetitions. I mean, if you did nine clean pull-ups and the tenth needed a tad of help, don't record all ten as if they all were done well. You should note the assisted repetition as only a half rep. If at one training session you rush between sets and then at the next session you take your time, you can't compare those two workouts evenly. You must be honest about details when entering data.

Indeed, your training diary should be more than just a list of exercises, sets, and reps. Many factors can be included in the journal. For instance, whether you intend to lose weight or not, monitoring your nutritional intake throughout the day is a reasonable move. In a few months, you will figure out the best foods to give you the best results.

If you are attempting to lose weight, it may be a good idea to monitor your body mass on a weekly basis. But please don't get into the useless habit of weighing yourself every day.

Also, record how many hours of sleep per night you are getting and how many times you wake in the night. Alternations in your sleep patterns may be a sign that your training load is too high.

Resting heart rate is a simple and workable indicator of your general physical wellbeing. A heart rate that's more than ten beats over your typical resting value is a sign of overtraining. But again, you need some stats.

Think of your training diary as a road map which is irreplaceable for keeping you on track for fitness success. With a detailed data, you will know what is working well for you and what doesn't. So, you can draw on when designing your future training programs.

Conclusion.

Fitness and general health are important parts of life. Good health is a result of a balanced lifestyle. Fitness should be a pleasant side of your life. There is nothing wrong with lifting weights. Actually, weights can be used for a variety of useful tricks. For example, you can pre-exhaust a particular muscle group before training a compound movement. I suppose it comes down to enjoying something and asking what you want from your workout. People who take up weight training usually more focused on building muscle mass and adding strength in certain movements. Calisthenics people are typically interested more in overall full-body strength than they are in increasing the size of isolated muscles. Both calisthenics and weight training contribute to general health and well-being. The best workout is the one that you actually will perform, remember?

Your real 'enemy at the gates' is a sedentary lifestyle. A sedentary lifestyle is a medical term used to describe a way of life with an excessive amount of daily sitting. Also, sedentary activities include lying, working the computer, watching TV, playing video games, and reading. Being inactive increases the risk of developing obesity, hypertension, cardiovascular disease, depression, anxiety, and premature aging.

Your genes, combined with your lifestyle choices, determine your health status. Our genes are virtually identical to those of our ancestors who lived here long ages ago. For them, daily physical activity was a necessary part of survival; it was not a lifestyle choice. In fact, today exercise is still essential for our general health and well-being. According to the Department of Health and Human Services, you need to be physically active for at least 150 minutes per week. Also, you should execute muscle-strengthening activities at least two days every week.

If you are sedentary, consult your physician before beginning any exercise regimen. It is never too late to make a change. Start with a light intensity aerobic activity that you enjoy. Gradually increase your level of activity each week until you reach optimal volume. Additionally to your aerobic exercise, start your muscle-strengthening program one day weekly, and gradually increase to more days.

So, calisthenics is about natural looking bodies, functional strength, building strong neurological connections to body, and creativity. Also, this is probably the most versatile of all workout styles. It seems that calisthenics is the future of fitness. By now it is evident there is a growing community of people who are committed to exercising with only the weight of their bodies and minimal equipment. You may join this community too!

Copyright © 2017 Timothy Morrison
All Rights Reserved.

You are not allowed to copy, modify, or sell this

content. No part of this book may be reproduced in

any form or by any means without prior written

permission of the copyright holder, excepting brief

quotes used in reviews.

DISCLAIMER: the author and the publisher do not
hold any responsibility for errors, omissions or
contrary interpretation of the subject matter herein.
This book is presented solely for motivational and
informational purposes only. Please consult a
physician before engaging in bodyweight training.

www.ingramcontent.com/pod-product-compliance
Lightning Source LLC
Chambersburg PA
CBHW071253280526
45788CB00004B/1701